Young, Dumb
&
Full of hmm...

I. R. Wright

Author: I. R. Wright
Editor: Stella Samuel

Keep an eye out for my new book:

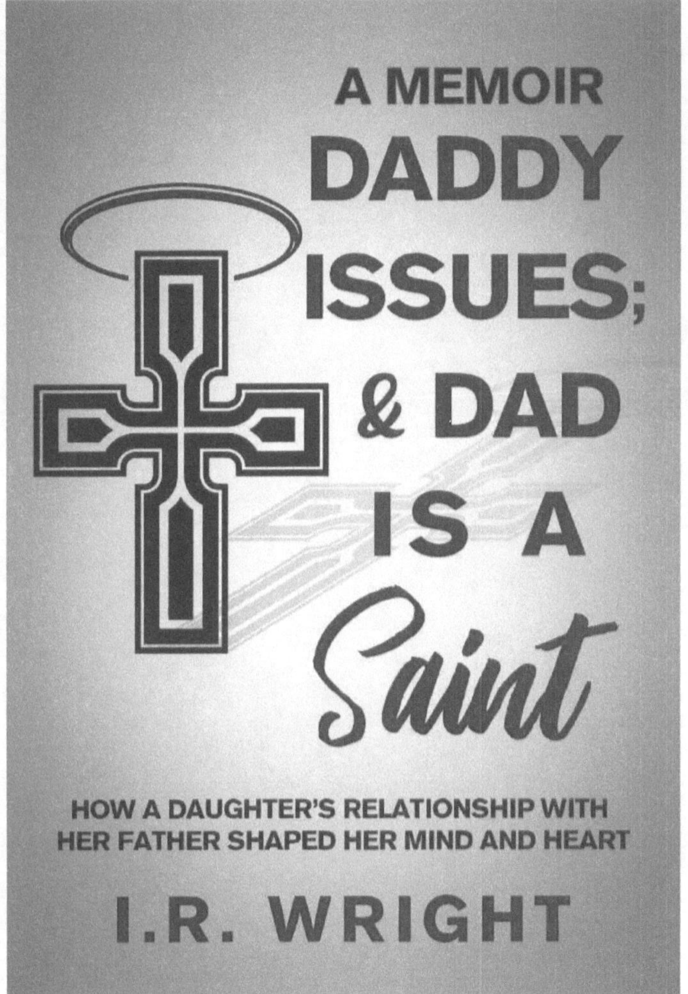

CONTENTS

<u>D is for Duke</u>: *the cop*

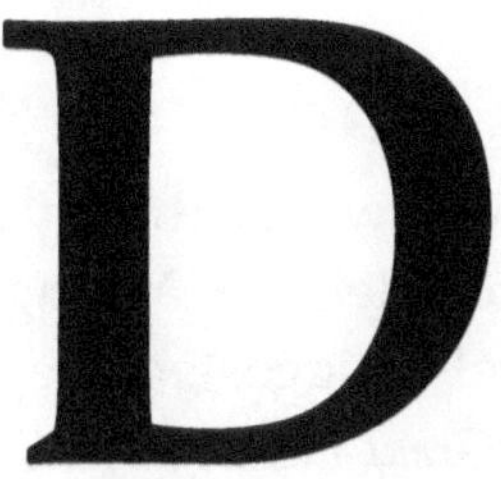is for Duke

—

Dating a cop. The man of my dreams, in my face.

Reality Star Twin: The Game
Reality Show: *Marrying the Game*
Why him: To me, The Game seemed like the perfect guy on the show. There were some arguments between him and his fiancé, Tiffney, but overall, he portrayed an image that his fiancé was the most important woman in his life.
Similarities to him: I always viewed Duke as a perfect guy. He was great when we were together. The only problem was when he left. His time away from me was a mystery. I didn't ever know what he did while away or why he was unavailable for my calls.

Duke was a low key easy going guy. Always down to do whatever I wanted to do, he somehow made every experience better, more enjoyable. Maybe he did this with ease because he was great eye candy. Or maybe because of the way he touched me when we were together. Or because he had a way of making me laugh. Either way, time with Duke was sure to be fun.

My relationship with Duke put simply… was fun. He didn't come with drama—only reasons to laugh and feel carefree. He was a friendly, happy person whose energy was contagious. He always gave me his undivided attention. He never used his cell phone when we were together, and that made me feel special and enriched the time we spent together.

Taking the Lead

During the summer of 2006, I turned twenty-three years old. I went out with a bunch of girlfriends to celebrate. Young, single, and ready to mingle. One of my friends suggested we go to a nightclub in New York City. *Of course! Great idea.* I loved dancing and flirting with guys in clubs. Exchanging numbers and making dates with hot men from the dance floor or bar was a specialty of mine.

My perspective on men had changed after the losers I'd dealt with before. I wanted a guy with charm and swag, but I had no room for disrespect. A man who knew how to treat me, who could offer a fun time, and give me respect was who I needed in my life. Any guy I dated had to come drama-free.

Manhattan was its usual bright noisy self as we walked from our cars to the club entrance. It was close to midnight but by the look of the traffic around us it could have been 5:00 p.m. The only distinguishing factor was the way people were dressed and the casualty with which they walked. My friends and I were all dressed scantly too with high heels and short dresses.

When we arrived at the club on the breathless summer night, I noticed a roped-off line with only a few people. The line led to a double entrance. One headed to the ground floor which had a restaurant and pool tables, and the other, off to the left, led to a flight of stairs going down to the dance floor. I started moving as soon as I heard the music before I even reached the bottom of the stairs. I sashayed in and danced around like I owned the place. My friends were right there with me. We were having a great time when I noticed a handsome gentleman lurking on the wall near a big speaker.

The basement level had a bar with lights so bright it was like looking into a solar eclipse given the contrast with the dark room. Huge speakers placed on either side of the bar made ordering drinks challenging. We couldn't talk over the music blasting, so I scanned the room for faces. Beautiful faces, familiar faces, anything to grab my attention. I caught his face by the big speaker away from the entrance.

I noticed him but reminded myself I was on a mission to have fun. I hoped he would make his way over to dance with me. The DJ played a song I loved, and I got lost dancing in the crowd before making my way back out to the speaker where my friends were hanging out.

I noticed him leave and come back to that spot near where we were all night. I kept wishing he would approach me, but he didn't. He didn't approach any of us. He just hung out near the speakers.

Since the club was dark, I couldn't see his face, but I liked his silhouette. I liked the way he wore his fitted Yankees hat, which he placed low on his head so it touched his eyebrows. I watched him walk and appreciated his football player physique. As the night wound down and the girls were ready to leave, I decided to get a better look at him. I needed to see if he was everything I thought he was. All the things I liked in a guy.

Making my way over to the speaker, I pretended I needed a break and sat down at a small table near there and checked him out. He noticed me looking and shot me a smile. I smiled back. *Oh yeah,* I thought. He's a cutie. I was hoping he'd walk over and spark up a conversation, but he stayed put. The music was loud, and he was right next to the speaker. I knew I wouldn't be able to say anything to him while he stood there. He wouldn't hear anything I said from where I was sitting either, but I didn't want to miss the opportunity to see him again. Desire to learn more about him built in me, and I had to come up with something quick.

In a swift move, I grabbed a napkin from the bar and asked for a pen. As fast as I could, I scribbled on the napkin and handed it to him. He looked puzzled when I handed him the napkin. Then he looked down at it and back at me before he laughed. That was not what I expected him to do. I had written a question I was hoping he would answer. Laughing was not a good sign. So, I took the napkin back and wrote again. "Maybe," I added to my original question of, "Do you like me? Circle Yes or No." *Let's try this again,* I thought. I walked over to where he was standing and handed him the napkin, then sat down again.

He kept laughing. In fact, he seemed to be laughing even harder. I couldn't decide if it was time to walk away or if something good might be coming. Besides, it was dark, and I couldn't make out much more of what his face might be trying to tell me.

"Yes," he said, nodding his head.

Yes, I thought to myself ecstatic he was interested. *Perfect!* It was time to go, so without delay, I handed him my phone so he could put his number in it, but he didn't. He reached into his pocket and instead he handed me his phone. *This is a great sign,* I thought. *He wants to be sure he can reach me. He wants the ball in his court.* I put my number in his phone and said goodbye, smiled and waved, then gave him a seductive walk to the exit. My girls were ready to go, and a few had already headed out. Two waited behind for me because they saw what I was up to with my napkin shenanigans.

Your Move

Duke called me the day after we met. When we spoke on the phone, we debated over who picked up who that night in the club.

"I noticed you first," Duke exclaimed. I almost heard his smile over the phone.

"If I never made my move, you would have let me leave," I shouted back with a huge smile.

"You don't know that! I was watching to make sure I didn't let you get away."

"Yeah, yeah."

Through our conversation, I learned Duke was an undercover police officer. He hadn't approached me that night because he was working. The club paid him to be in the room to ensure nothing bad happened or rather to handle any situation quickly and appropriately. That made me feel better. So maybe he did like me, and I wasn't too crazy for making the first move to talk to him.

Finding out Duke was a police officer was a major turn on for me. He was the only guy I noticed that night in the club, and he was all of my favorite things—tall, dark, and handsome. Born and raised in Brooklyn, he had a smooth New York swag when he walked. Best of all were his dark eyes, trimmed with beautiful dark eyebrows. Combined with his skin tone I had no chance when looking at his eyes. They never seemed to open fully and made him seem like he was of Asian descent. He had a big strong frame that looked like it belonged to a football player. And he carried a gun. Legally. Not only was he cute, but I knew I would be completely safe around him. He would always protect me.

"So, when are you going to let me take you out?" He asked.

I didn't want to delay. We had met over the weekend, and I wanted to see him as soon as possible. We went back and forth and realized the next time we were both free was the following Wednesday. The middle of the week on a workday was not ideal, but I was sure it would be worth it.

"Okay, I'll see you then," I said hanging up the phone.

Trying to Lasso the Moon

For our first date, Duke came out to see me in my hometown. We were excited to see each other again and didn't care to work out specific details of what we would do once he arrived. The only plan we made was to go to a local spot. A fun evening at an indoor amusement park of sorts. With games, pool, bowling, and more, we figured we'd decide what to do once we got there.

"There are so many trees," Duke said when he called me to let me know he had gotten off the highway and was close. "Are there no trees in Brooklyn?" I asked playfully. He sounded astonished, so I was happy he'd found a sense of wonder before the date started. *We're off to a great start,* I thought. "I'm outside," he said.

I made my way out. It was summer, so I dressed for the weather. With little on, I grabbed my bag and walked down the two flights of stairs in front of my mother's house as cute as possible and got in his car.

I was living with my mother at the time. She had remodeled her house and had room for me again. I was no longer enjoying living with my dad as Aunt Becky moved back in and living there got uncomfortable.

"You look nice," he said as I sat down.

"Thank you."

"Now where to?"

"Drive straight down the block and make a left," I said.

"Are you hungry?" he asked before we made it to the end of the short block. "I just started feeling hungry all of a sudden."

"Okay. We can grab something to eat on the way. Let me know if you see something that looks good."

As we drove, I checked him out while trying to make sure I didn't miss any of our turns. We saw a pizza place on our route and decided to stop. I noticed his outfit when we got out the car. A nice navy-blue polo shirt with blue jeans around his waist. That impressed me because most guys wore their jeans below their butts.

Duke looked clean and polished. I wondered if he had his gun on him. It didn't matter because I felt safe in his presence. His broad shoulders made me feel protected all by themselves. We ordered our pizzas and sat at a bar facing the street while we tried to look discreet checking each other out. We shot each other flirtatious smiles when caught looking at one another but didn't talk much because we were stuffing our mouths.

"Okay. So." I stood up as I made my way over to the garbage to throw out my plate. "The place is just a few minutes from here."

"Cool," Duke said standing up as well. "Let's go."

He pushed the shop door open with one hand and stood back so I could walk out. I grinned as I graciously passed him. We made our way back to his car, and he walked over to the passenger's side to open the door for me. I appreciated every little gesture and had the feeling of melting in happiness with each action. The date hadn't officially started, and I already felt very special.

When we arrived at the plaza, I walked Duke around

showing him different things we could do. We decided to bowl first. I wasn't overly excited about bowling, but I was happy to spend time with him. After paying to play and getting some shoes, Duke set up the scorecard with our names. I took my time walking around the alley searching for the perfect ball before sitting down to change my shoes. He was cute. I hid my huge smile each time I stole a glance. I played my own version of hard to get. While I changed shoes, Duke walked around to find his bowling ball. He came back with the heaviest ball he could find.

"Okay, Killa," I said mocking him with a sweet smile. I imagined him strutting over to our lane and dropping the ball just before ending up in the next lane where someone else was playing. I giggled. *Why do guys always want the 15-pound balls?*

Not long after we started bowling, we were full on flirting.

"Okay, not bad," I said smiling at him. His first spin knocked down seven pins.

"The light got in my eye. I normally get all ten," he said smiling and rubbing his eyes. "Plus, I think you're trying to distract me with that beautiful smile."

I smiled a sweet smirk and said, "That's alright. You'll get 'em next time." I held up both hands for a double high-five. Operation hard to get fell apart as I melted for his charm.

My turn was next. *Bang* was the sound as all ten pins went down. He looked up in shock, but he was clearly impressed. I was in shock too but didn't want him to know. I played it cool like I bowl all the time.

"I know this is our first date, so I wanted to be a gentleman and not beat you. But I see you have skills, so I'm going to show you how to play for real now." A flirtatious yet competitive smile spread across his face.

Another group started their game in the lane next to us.

"Watch my shoes," Duke whispered to me laughing, suggesting the new guests might take them. Each time he smiled at me, I felt closer to him.

I don't remember who won the first game, but after Duke knocked down any pins, I made of point of giving him a high five or two. Even when he got gutter balls, I gave him high fives to say it's okay. It was fun to touch him, so either way, I was winning. The longer we played the more we grew comfortable with one another. Then the trash talking started.

The whole night was filled with Duke's antics. I laughed the whole game, and by the end of the second game, I didn't care who'd won the games. It was just as much fun losing as winning. Duke had fun too, and once we finished bowling both games, we weren't ready to leave one another.

The bowling alley had a bar that seemed like the best option for us to continue our evening. It was a way to stay together and feel each other out. Get to know each other a little more in person. It was a Wednesday after all so, we probably should have wrapped up the night, but instead, we headed to the bar. *One little drink can't hurt.*

We sat down at a table across from the bar and talked more. The flirting remained consistent between us. Duke noticed an air hockey table just a few feet from us and asked if I was interested in playing.

"I'd love to," I said. It didn't take long for us to get rowdy. Duke was either trying really hard to win or was too strong for the game because his puck kept flying off the table. I was surprised when it happened the first time and almost fell out laughing. Maybe Duke wanted me to laugh more or just wanted to win, I'm not sure but he continued to do it. Every time it happened, I laughed harder and harder. All the noise we made brought over a few kids from the bowling alley eager to play.

We finished our last game and gave them the table when Duke asked, "Would you like another drink?"

I didn't think before saying, "Yes." Even though it was a Wednesday, it was still early, and I was having fun. So, no way did I want the date to end. We sat down at the tables again and talked about nothing while still flirting. Then, after a while, Duke looked at his watch and asked, "Do you need to head out?"

"No, I've got time."

"Let's go do something else in here. I noticed miniature golf when we came in. Do you want to do that?"

"Yeah, let's go."

We left the bowling alley and headed down two flights of escalators to the miniature golf courses. To our disappointment, they were closed. It was the middle of the week and later than we realized. I thought Duke might suggest we wrap it up and head home, but he was unfazed by the late hour. He wanted to do something else, if I was up for it, of course.

"The pool hall was still open when we left the bowling alley. Do you want to do that instead?" He asked.

I hated playing pool, but I was looking forward to spending more time with Duke. "Yeah, that sounds fun," I said partially lying as we headed back up the escalator. "Let's do that."

But Wait, There's More

The plaza was a ghost town. No one lingered around. We saw only one other couple in the pool hall when we got there.

"Are you guys about to close?" Duke asked when we walked in.

"No, you guys are good to play if you want," the attendant told us.

"Sweet." Duke paid to get us a table, and we were off.

Pool can be a seductive physical game. We didn't miss the opportunity to connect. Duke wrapped his strong arms around me with the excuse of helping me improve my stroke. I moved the pool stick between my fingers back and forth knowing he was watching. I loved every minute of it.

"Alright. Now, pay attention," he said smiling. "This is how you do it."

We graduated from the high-fives we had been giving each other while bowling to hugging one another to congratulate a job well done.

"Oh! Great job!" I said while extending my arms and walking toward him after a good shot.

"Thank you," he said with a smile hugging me back. "Your

hair really looks beautiful."

"Thank you," I said. I tried to focus on my shot but was distracted by my desire to be closer to him. "Watch out!" I screamed as I hit a ball off the table. It was my turn to be excited doing a bit too much. Duke was a great sport picking up my balls and making jokes about my mistakes.

He said funny things like, "Don't make me have to arrest you. This is starting to seem like assault with a deadly weapon." Well, he was less corny and more charming, but the jokes kept coming.

I enjoyed being with him but don't really care for pool, so when that game was over, I didn't want to play another. I liked my time with him and didn't want it to end, but I needed to get out of the pool hall. Just as we made our way out, Duke noticed the indoor arcade.

"Oh, they have video games in there?" he said as he gazed in.

I was feeling all the lyric's to P!nk's song *Glitter in the Air*, thinking about what might happen next. *Is he going to want to go in? Do I look desperate if I go in with him rather than wrapping the night up? Should I be playing harder to get? This guy seems like a nice catch, and I don't want him to write me off after tonight. I thought I should go, but I desperately wanted him to ask me into the arcade.* I paused but would follow him in if he wanted. No hesitation. I didn't want to lose the sensation he gave me. I was so happy. Everything was going great, and I didn't want it to stop. *Please, please, ask me to join you in the arcade.*

"So, I know it's late but, do you want to check out the arcade for a bit?"

YES! I thought. But I said, "Sure, let's do it." I tried to say it as cool as possible.

But Wait. That's Not All. There's More.

We walked into the arcade checking out the different games. I tried to find a 'date night' kind of game when I stumbled upon a photo booth. I had a flip phone at the time and no ability to capture pictures on it. The photo booth would be a great way to capture the memory of the night and see my handsome guy's face once he left. I wondered if he'd want to do it and hoped suggesting it wouldn't ruin the experience and make me seem thirsty.

"Let's take a picture," I blurted it out before I could stop myself. The risk was worth it.

"Really? Of course, let's do it."

We smiled and posed checking ourselves out on the screen as the camera flashed. It was a fail. I was disappointed when the pictures printed out. I looked terrible, and Duke felt the same about himself. That didn't stop me from keeping the picture. I smiled as I dropped it in my bag. It was still a fun memory and captured our first date. *Who knows where this relationship might go. I might need this for our wedding reel.*

Off to the next thing. We walked around more. I was willing to play any game as long as it meant more time with Duke. And that was exactly what we did. Played a few of the games. The games spouted tickets we could redeem for prizes. The only prizes we wanted was time together, so we gave all our tickets to a few kids hanging out. Then, enough was enough, and it was time for us to let go and head out. We had done a lot for our first date, and even though I wasn't quite ready to wrap it up, it was time. I didn't want to embarrass myself and try to drag out the night, so I swallowed my feelings and hoped we would have another exciting experience together some other time.

We walked back to Duke's car without talking. I put my head down and pulled myself together. *Relax*, I thought. *Don't be sad.* Duke made a discovery and was about to give us one last chance to spend some more time together.

"I really want to see Superman in 3D. Have you seen it?"

Huh? I thought. *Okay, I guess he's planning the next date already.* I was tired, and my whole go with whatever he said routine was wearing off. "No, I'm not much of a Superman fan." I didn't worry about ruining our next date by being honest. I figured he was into me, but my brain slowed with exhaustion.

"3D movies are great! Would you be interested in checking it out? You won't be disappointed."

I heard him, but he seemed to mumble. I looked up and saw the movie theater with a poster for Superman and got a quick boost of energy. "Now?" *Um, wake up dumb-dumb. He's found a way for us to spend more time together. Don't blow it.* "Yes, sure. I am down to check it out."

"All right. Let's do it," he said. So, we headed for the movie theater. This meant locking in a decent amount of time together in the dark. It was after midnight and a little cuddling seemed like a good idea.

He Loves Me?

I loved the way we both looked in our 3D shades. The shades were silly but still cute. I expected to have glasses with one eye red and one eye blue, but these were different. They didn't look exactly like sunglasses but were very close. I was excited to match with Duke. *Glasses Twins!* I could already see us color coordinating outfits like Jay-Z and Beyoncé with their boots in the '03 *Bonnie & Clyde* video. The 3D glasses made us look like we were early movers on new cool eyeglasses. *Couples match, right? So, we were almost an official couple.*

"These glasses are cool," I said to Duke.

"Yeah, I was expecting blue and red glasses."

"Me too. I'm happy I wasn't alone." We both laughed and looked into each other's eyes. Duke grabbed my hand, and we headed to the theater.

We found a seat in the middle and sat down. There weren't many people sharing the theater with us. If I had to guess, there were maybe five others. I assumed most rational people were home sleeping, so they'd be refreshed for work the next day. We had the whole row to ourselves as well as a few behind and in front of us.

After the movie started and had been playing for a while, Duke grabbed my hand and kissed it. Sounds sweet, but he did it in the most seductive way causing an eruption inside my body. His soft lips on top of my hand were the last straw on the camel's back for the chemistry we had been building between us. I was overwhelmed by his presence and our energy together. My insides melted even more than they had been all night, and I was more intrigued by him. I wondered how he did that. A simple kiss on the hand had never been so sensual. Maybe it was a side effect from the two drinks we'd had earlier. Or from the fatigue starting to settle in.

A little later he leaned over and kissed me. His lips were as soft as they were on my hand, and he was gentle with his touch. The kiss was simple but sexy. His fatigue must have kicked in as well. The next time he touched me, it was his head hitting mine as we dozed off together. The temperature in the theater dropped, and in my fatigue, I was freezing. My sexy summer top and skirt were no match for the theater's air conditioning system. Duke didn't have any extra layers with his outfit either.

In the early hours of the morning, we drove back to my mother's house and sat out front in his car and talked. "You looked really beautiful tonight," Duke whispered. As I pulled out my keys indicating I was about to go inside, he touched both sides of my face and said, "I had a good time with you tonight." He leaned in with a smile, kissed me, and then said, "Good night."

Our Time Together

Duke and I had a few more magical and wonderful dates after our first, but there was a problem. I noticed a pattern when we weren't together. He would disappear. Sometimes it was because he was working. Understandable, of course. Sometimes it was because he was hanging out with his friends. Understandable as well. Reflecting on anytime we spent together, I always had his undivided attention. So, I couldn't really be upset. He was a present person. He lived in the moment which was one factor that made our time together so enjoyable.

In time, being unavailable unless we were together wore on me. He would tell me he'd call me later when he left his friends and never did. I hated it, and it happened often. I often felt he'd say those things to get me off the phone. Given my background dating guys who said they would do something and didn't, I held his words against his integrity and began to trust him less. I didn't like how he said he would do something then didn't do it. He'd eventually call back when the timing was right for him. I was so crazy about him and couldn't resist talking to him and seeing him again.

On one of these occasions, I called Duke only to hear him say he was busy hanging out with friends. I heard his friends laughing and joking in the background. "Okay," I said.

"I'm going to call you later," he said. But I knew he wouldn't, and it frustrated me. He said those things all too often knowing he wouldn't honor it.

"Listen, you always say you're going to call back and you don't."

"I'm sorry," he said. "I promise, I'm going to call you later, but I've got to go now."

Wow, promise. Okay, he must be serious this time.

That night, I kept my phone close. I knew he'd call because, this time, he promised. He had never *promised* to call me back before. He understood how much it hurt when he hadn't called me back in the past, and this time, he knew how important that promise was. He would call me back. I knew the difference between telling me and promising me. But, that night, he never called. I was done with men who lied and didn't keep their word, so I was done with Duke. To help myself remember the pain that comes from a man who lies all the time, I changed Duke's name in my phone to Bobby. I knew seeing "Bobby" calling me would be a major turn off, and I would not answer the phone. I closed the door on any possibilities for a future with Duke.

Ghost of Bobby

The day I changed his name in my phone, I hung out with a few girlfriends at a local restaurant. That night, the restaurant turned into a club and hosted a party. My friends were invited by their friends, so pretty much everyone in the spot knew each other.

Duke finally had time to call me back and gave me a ring.

When I saw "Bobby" on my caller ID, I hit the ignore button and kept dancing and drinking. Losing myself in the music as I often did, I enjoyed the evening up to that point. I'm not sure why but Duke called right back, but I hit ignore again and danced some more. Duke must have had some free time and maybe even wanted to see me because he kept calling. I kept hitting ignore. I wanted him to know I wasn't going to answer.

After about the fifteenth call, a guy friend of mine noticed what I was doing and looked over my shoulder to see who I was hanging up on. "Are you dating Bobby?" he asked.

I was embarrassed that he knew Bobby and more embarrassed about having his name in my phone. It associated me with him. Before I responded to his question, he continued. "I know he's a real jerk. My sister dated him, so I understand why you're not picking up."

In an instant, memories flooded my mind, and I wondered if we were dating him at the same time. "I dated him before, but I am not dating him now. When did your sister date him?" I asked. Then I stopped myself. "Actually, forget it. This is someone else."

That was enough for me to change Duke's name in my phone back from Bobby to Duke. I still had a soft spot for him in my heart, and since he'd called all night, I knew he was sorry and was trying to show me as much. I ended up speaking to him later because he kept calling me. I couldn't resist answering when I saw his name. He was not Bobby. Bobby was something else, and no one deserved to be thought of as Bobby. Except of course, Bobby.

The Good Thing About Strippers

While I had some great dates and even more fun with Duke, it was months before we had sex. At the seven month mark after meeting, we finally did it. We started out the night at a local club. I was with my friends, and Duke and a friend of his met us there. He was really sweet to my friends and offered to buy them all drinks. We were hanging out and having fun when someone suggested we make our way to a local strip club.

Once we arrived, Duke noticed the club had security and metal detectors. Since Duke had his gun on him, he needed to speak to the bouncers in private to let them know he was a cop and carrying. They were fine with it and let him right in without paying. I was impressed and proud to be with a man who had the respect of the bouncers. He got bonus safety points for wearing a gun. I was safe. Protected.

We had so much fun in that club. Not only was Duke my personal body guard, he also was generous and attentive. There were about six of us, and we all sat at the bar together. Duke didn't have cash on him, so he went to the ATM inside the club for cash. That particular machine should have had a sign that read "SUCKER" because anyone who went into a strip club without cash was about to get exploited financially. There was a charge of almost $10 to withdraw money compared to other standard ATM fees of two to three dollars.

Once he got his cash out, the bartender gave him singles so we could tip the performers as they danced nearby. He shared his singles with our whole crew. He even offered to buy everyone drinks and kept finding ways to make me feel special. As the bartender propped her boobs up on the bar to ask what Duke wanted to drink, he turned to me and locked eyes before looking back at her to order our drinks.

Sitting at the bar meant we had front row seats to the ladies who danced on poles at both ends of the bar and the girls free-styling in the middle of the bar without poles. Since we were tipping, additional ladies walked in the bartender's area to get close and do special performances to get our dollars. The show was spectacular.

I studied their moves in awe of the dancers. They had incredible talent, and I wanted to do each move for Duke once we got home to my place. One lady climbed to the top of the pole then flipped upside down and danced as she slid down the pole slowly. *Okay*, I thought watching and committing her moves to memory. *Left cheek, left cheek, left cheek, right.* Another girl stopped right in front of us and played with herself. *Not impressed*, I thought as an older man pushed past me to give her money. Another dancer got on the pole and swung around before beginning her routine. She did a bump and grind going down the pole with total control.

During all this, Duke made me feel like I was the best thing in the entire club. Of all the times we had gone out, he was never more all over me than there. He could not keep his hands and lips off me, which made me feel good. While he could have been watching the dancers strip, he was sticking his tongue down my throat. After hanging out for a few hours I decided we had been there long enough, and it was time to go.

Cops are Safe

Duke did not want to use condoms during intercourse. At this point, after having dating Chuck and my intimidation over speaking up, I didn't hold back. Certain I wanted to use condoms, I let him know I was uncomfortable having sex without one. I made it clear I wanted him to wear one.

"What do you want to use a condom for? I'm a cop. We get tested for HIV every six months. I'm safe."

"I would feel more comfortable using a condom. We're not in an exclusive relationship."

"You don't want to use those things. Trust me."

I insisted, but he pushed back. He touched me in ways that made me forget I had ever asked. Talk about young and dumb. *Okay, just this one time. But next time, we need to use a condom.* He never did, and I never made him. Reflecting on what I was doing, made me cry. I wasn't in a committed relationship with Duke. I didn't want to have a baby with him. But I didn't know how to make him put on a condom. I didn't try hard enough either.

I felt strongly I wanted to have protected sex and had an internal conflict that got stronger every time he disappeared. *What was I doing? What if I got pregnant? The baby would certainly be cute if it looked like him. But, really, what would I do if I got pregnant? Would I keep it? Would he love it? What if the baby looked like me? Would he hate it like I felt like my dad sometimes hated me? What was I doing?* I needed to make a change, but I couldn't resist his embrace. I wouldn't fight his desires despite mine.

A Return to Getting Dumber

Most often, I spent time with Duke at my house or near it. Every time he invited me to his house or to hang out with him around his house, we had drama. The worst instance was when he invited me to join him at a BBQ in Brooklyn at his cousin's house. After making the almost hour-long drive from my place to get there, I was a little intimidated about going in because there were lots of people in the yard. I didn't know anyone but Duke. After more than a year of dating, it would be my first time meeting his family. A big move. I wanted to do it, but I was scared. My fear was so deep, I delayed leaving home for more than an hour trying to hype myself up for the experience while also trying to relax my fears.

I had met one of his cousins briefly on another trip out to see him, and he made some strange comments that threw me off. I didn't hear what he said, but by the tone, he seemed like he was being fresh with me. When I asked him to repeat himself, Duke shut him down and told him not to speak to me again. We were dropping him off at his house, so he rode in silence until we got there, and he got out. *What was I going to say if he was there tonight and said something slick, or what if someone else said something to me? How would I handle it?* I wanted to get their stamp of approval and earn more cool points with Duke.

When I arrived at the BBQ, Duke came out to meet me at my car and said there had been a change of plans. We would be leaving instead of staying at the BBQ. I was relieved I didn't have to meet several new people at one time. I would have preferred to meet them in smaller groups to start. I also knew his mother was present, and I wanted to be sure I made a good impression on her. Now, I didn't have to worry about that. Since we were leaving soon, there was no need for me to get out of the car. I wasn't meeting anyone at all. We didn't leave right then because he needed to take his mother and brother home, and he didn't want to rush them out. His little brother was playing, and his mom was finishing a drink.

"They live in the projects. Are you afraid to drive into the projects in Brooklyn?" he asked me half laughing but wanting to be sure I would be okay with the plan.

"Should I be afraid?" I countered. "I would prefer to live a little longer, and I like my car without bullet holes."

I didn't understand why he had me wait in the car, but I was so wrapped up in his cuteness, I had a hard time thinking straight around him. I didn't think I had wasted my time driving out because after all, I was with Duke. That meant a lot to me.

He kissed me and said, "Let me run inside and see if they are ready."

I admired Duke's physique as he walked away. He was as handsome as ever with his broad shoulders, beautiful eyes, and fly swag. He smiled at me one last time before disappearing into the yard. I looked forward to our time alone and turned up my radio to get me in the mood. My phone rang and pulled me out of the moment for a second. It was my sister. One of my favorite people.

"Hello?" I said.

"Hey. What are you doing?"

"In Brooklyn about to hang out with Duke. What about you?" My sister had met Duke a few weeks back at a bowling outing we did with a bunch of my friends.

"Oh, okay. That's nice," she said. "I wasn't calling you for anything just to say, 'Hi.'"

"Okay. I'm waiting for him to come outside so I can talk to you in the meantime." My sister and I talked mindlessly for a while before Duke appeared again. "Oh, he's back. Let me go. I'll talk to you later," I said then hung up the phone.

He hopped into the car again. I was confused because I thought he would just be coming by to let me know we were leaving. Nevertheless, I was happy he was next to me because I could get more kisses.

"Hey. Why are you getting into my car? They are still not ready?" I asked.

"No. It should just be a little while now," he said and then changed the subject. "You know I really care about you, right? I care about you much more than you realize. So, I want you to know just how much I care about you." He kept repeating himself.

"I care about you, too," I said.

"Okay, but I really, really care about you. I need you to know you are very special to me. I don't think you realize how special you are to me." He leaned over and kissed me.

His words were touching. It was the first time he'd said anything like that to me. I wondered what brought about his sentiments. Why he wanted to say these things to me. Was he trying to tell me he loved me?

We stopped kissing, and he looked me deep in my eyes. "I really, really care about you." At this point, his mother had left the yard and stood in front of the driveway looking at us. "Oh, that's my mom. She must be ready," he said. "Let me go see if my brother is ready to go." And he was gone again.

I called my sister back to chat with her while I passed the time, but our conversation took an unexpected turn.

"Wow. So, he just got you sitting outside waiting for him, huh?" she asked.

"He's waiting for his mom and brother," I said. I found him to be a considerate person. He never rushed me, and I couldn't see him rushing his mom or other family members when they were having a good time and he wanted to leave.

"So, you're just going to sit outside of a BBQ and wait for him?" she asked.

"Well, he said he was coming soon," I rationalized.

"We were on the phone for almost an hour, so I know you've been waiting out there longer than that. If you're willing to just sit in your car and wait for him, then do that. I would not let a man treat me the way you're letting him treat you. But if that's the way you want to live your life, if that's the way you want to be treated by guys…"

Those words hit like a wake-up call. I didn't realize how much time had passed since we got on the phone. I enjoyed my conversation with her without thinking about the time passing, and I was happy to be seeing Duke soon. But she was absolutely right. I did not want anyone to treat me like that.

Her last words hit hard. I tried to breathe deep as my sister's words knocked the breath out of me. "If that's the way you want to be treated by guys… It's your life, do what you want, but stop calling me to complain about waiting for this guy when you're choosing to live your life as a loser. He's not picking you, and you seem to be happy about that. Hence, why you're sitting there…"

Without thinking, I started my car and drove off without looking back to see if Duke had come out ready to leave. *How could I be so dumb?* I felt terrible. *Why did it take my sister's words for me to see that this was happening to me? For me to realize the ludicrousness of what I was doing.* I kept listening to my wise, younger sister as I drove off. She pulled me from under Duke's spell with every word. "…you can do what you want. Just know I'm not sitting on the phone with you to help you pass the time."

"You're right," I said. "And I just pulled off. Thank you for helping me pull it together." We hung up.

But He's Really Sorry

I wasn't gone ten minutes when Duke called me. He was frantic.

"Where are you?" he screamed into the phone.

"I left!" I screamed back. "I just realized you had me waiting outside for an hour and a half!" I hung up the phone. He called me right back. I didn't answer. And he called me again.

"I'm sorry!" he screamed when I answered. "Please, come back!"

"You are making me feel really dumb!" I yelled back.

"You can't leave! I'm so sorry," he said. "I really care about you. You just don't get it. Come back. We are about to leave now. I'm so sorry. Come back. Where are you? Did you get on the highway yet? Come back. PLEASE, come back. Please! I'm sorry." I looked at the highway but felt a tug at my heart. I didn't want to leave him, especially not after waiting all that time to be with him.

He continued to beg. I had never heard him beg and plead like he did that day. I'm not sure what went wrong to make him treat me like that, but he was clearly sorry. I really loved spending time with Duke and felt torn with him on the phone in hysterics. He was always calm, cool, and collected. *No harm in second chances. They were ready to leave, so no more waiting. I'm already here, so I should enjoy tonight. I've earned it.* I turned my car around and drove back without any idea where I was going. *Is this my turn?* I thought as I weaved in and out of the Brooklyn streets lost. *He better be ready when I get back because this is too much.*

Getting More Dumb Again

He called me back to make sure I wasn't heading home.

"Where you at?"

"I'm lost."

"What do you see…" He gave me directions over the phone to get back to the BBQ.

Once I was back in front of the house, there was no sight of Duke. I expected to see him getting into the car with his mother and brother when I arrived. I sent him a text to say I was there.

Okay, we're about to come out now, he wrote back.

I waited patiently. Fifteen minutes went by before I lost my cool and left again. This time I was really done. Done with him. Done with trying to hang out with him. I didn't care that I drove all the way out there and wasted two hours of my life sitting in my car. There was no chance I wanted anything else to do with him.

Duke called me after I got about three blocks away, only about five minutes after I left. He was hysterical again and asking where I was. He said he was in the car with his mom and brother driving to drop them off.

"I'm going home," I stated with determination.

"Why? I'm in the car. Meet me at my place." He was hysterical doing a bad job of trying to contain himself in front of his mother and brother.

"I'm going home. I can't believe you made me wait again. I know you're upset, and that's okay. We won't be hanging out anymore."

Looking back at the situation now, I can say I think Duke invited me out and then someone else showed up. Someone who he didn't want to see us together. Maybe it was an ex or a current fling. Maybe he balanced his time between both of us by going back inside and coming outside to be with me.

For the life of me, I cannot understand how I didn't see that at the time. I was way too into him and way too excited about spending time with him. And, I was far too relieved about not meeting his whole family and all his friends in one sitting.

Further, in reflection, I realize all his "I care about you" statements were his internal struggle in deciding who he would spend the night with. His behaviors told me he chose me over the other girl at the BBQ.

He Loves Me Not

I put up with Duke's shit time and time again. He would stay away just long enough for us to have a mental reset from all the hurt, pain, and drama that last separated us. Once, he lost my number, or deleted it, and reach out to one of my girlfriends, Samantha, to get it. She was in touch with him through his friend who she met the night we all went to the strip club. When she asked if it was okay to give him my number, I lit up inside at the thought of him. I heard Duke's name and almost felt my heart smile.

"Yes," I said. "You can give it to him."

Whenever he felt like it, Duke would hit me up with a text out of the blue. Though time had passed, it didn't feel like it to me. No other guy I dated in between our time apart gave my heart the pleasure I got from Duke. The time that passed only worked in his favor. It made me forget the bad experiences. A flood of positive memories ran through me anytime I thought of him or heard from him. I only remembered all the great things about him. His swag. How he touched me. His physique. His beautiful eyes. He was the man of my dreams.

Duke texted me one Valentine's Day saying 'Hey.' Once we started chatting, he made it perfectly clear he only hit me up because he was horny, not because he was looking to be romantic or do anything romantic with me. Somehow, he ended up in my bed that night. I'm sure he cleaned up the statement afterwards with something like 'I'm not trying to be rude, I'm just being honest' or some other nonsense. I loved being with him so much, what he said and how he meant it didn't matter. I wanted to enjoy the moment. The draw and excitement of hanging out with Duke outweighed my logic every time he called.

I know how it must look. There couldn't be anything this man should have been able to say or do to rectify a comment like that. And that's correct. But everybody plays the fool, right? I mean, maybe it's a role I've played a couple of times, but am I the only one? Haven't most women suffered from good dick disease? From a good guy. You know, a good-looking guy with a job. No kids. His own place. His own car? His type was slim pickings where I lived.

It gets worse. While prepping for this book, I read several journal entries from our time together and lost my breath gasping when I read about the time he left me stranded at an airport after telling me he was going to come and pick me up. I don't remember all the details of the story, and I didn't write them in the journal. I do know there was no Uber at the time, and I don't remember ever taking a taxi from the airport. So, I must have called a family member to pick me up. Even worse was that he didn't call or text me to say he wasn't coming. He just didn't show up and didn't respond to my calls or texts while I was waiting for him at our agreed upon time at the airport. This huge red flag was not enough to get me to stop dating Duke. It may have led to a break, but I went back after that too.

Looking back on this relationship, I see how much I ignored the truth or didn't care to pay attention to it in exchange for fun. From hanging out in my car for hours at BBQs to ignoring derogatory comments. I should have had more respect for myself than to allow everything Duke did. But in retrospect, I can honestly say I had fun with him every time we hung out. And when I wasn't having fun with him, I walked away, even if I couldn't stay away. Possibly, those absences made my heart grow fonder of him, which was an unintended consequence.

He Played Me

Duke and I had been dating off and on for about three years when I got a call from my doctor's office while at work.

"I have some bad news for you," she said. "We got back your pap smear, and you have HPV."

"What's that?" I asked.

"Well, right now, it's not a major issue, but it's been known to cause cancer among other health issues…." My heart stopped. I stopped listening. I needed to call Duke right away. "… can you come in for a follow up appointment…" Everything was a blur. I ended that call as fast as I could and ran into the bathroom with my cell phone.

"Hello?"

"I have HPV," I whispered before crying hysterically.

"Hey. Don't cry," he said "It's not that big of a deal. The doctors try to make it seem like a big deal, but it's not. You're going to be fine, and I am one hundred percent here for you."

"I could get cancer!" I whispered and cried even harder.

"Don't cry," he said. "I'm here for you. If you need anything at all, you can call me I'm here for you. It's really not that big of a deal. Listen. I'm at work now and need to get of this phone. I will give you a call later, but you have nothing to worry about, and you don't have to cry. I am here for you. Okay?"

I hung up and stayed in the bathroom for twenty minutes crying about everything the doctor said to me. *The possibility of death for a man I wasn't even in a relationship with… Never having kids, having complicated pregnancies. For what? I now have all this to deal with for what? What do I have to show for it?* I was inconsolable. Lucky for me, no one from my office came into the bathroom because it was really small with only two stalls, so I would have been busted.

I hoped he would call to check on me that night after my hysterical phone call to him, but he didn't. I waited over the weekend hoping he would reach out to check on me, but he didn't call then either. He never called to see if I was okay. After my HPV diagnosis and lack of concern from Duke, I reached a point of no return for our relationship. I didn't want anything to do with him. I never spoke to him again after that teary-eyed phone call.

The Silver Lining

I learned some powerful lessons through my time with Duke.
1. How being present makes life more fulfilling
2. That it's important to hear and not just listen
3. About knowing and speaking your truth
4. To live your truth at any consequence

When I was with Duke, I always had his full attention. He wasn't the type to check his cell phone or do anything but have fun and give me his undivided attention. It made me feel like I was important to him and increased the fun in hanging out with him.

Good listening skills help make all relationships better, so I work to ensure I'm listening to everyone around me now, not just hearing what they say. But listening for their needs and true understanding rather than skewing reality to believe it's fulfilling my own agenda.

I know I always heard what Duke said, but I wasn't always listening. I thought he was the salt of the earth. The best thing ever. In my head, when I talked to him, all I heard him say was 'Let's have some fun!' When we made plans to hang out, all I could think about was how much fun we were going to have together. In my head, I was in a real relationship with him. I attribute that disconnection from reality to how much I worked.

I had taken a full-time job at the magazine where I was previously temping which had a lot of responsibilities and took up a lot of my time. I had also started a part-time job while taking language classes. My romantic life was not a huge priority. There wasn't much time to focus on it. I did what made me happy. I didn't realize how inconsistent my time was with Duke. It took a comment from a girlfriend of mine for me to realize how much he wasn't around. The bigger problem was I was falling in love with him in our spare time dates.

A guy who called me on Valentine's Day of all days and flat out told me he just called because he was horny, should never have had a chance to say anything else. While I was having casual sex with guys for convenience, Duke was more than a casual exchange. He was my dream. I was a casual experience for him. The disconnection to my romantic life from my personal and business lives had created a conflict in my decision making and ultimately left me heartbroken. I was having casual unprotected sex with a man who was probably having casual unprotected sex with other women and passing around HPV to all of us. If I had been clear that I was having convenient sex with Duke, I would have made him wrap it up with no question.

OKAY SO, HOW WAS IT? READY FOR MORE?

GET THE FULL BOOK
SEARCH FOR:
YOUNG, DUMB & FULL OF HMM…

OR JUST THE NEXT CHAPTER:

- Daddy's Love Lessons
- First Teenage Love Affair
- Dating a F- Boy
- Dating an Older Man
- Dating a NYC Cop
- Dating a Cute Thug
- Dating a Nerdy Nudist
- Full Book: Young, Dumb & Full of hmm…

Thank you for taking the time to read this Chapter! Was it what you expected? Something you think other people would enjoy?

I humbly and kindly ask that you please provide a review of this book. Share your thoughts to help others know what you experienced while reading this.

I am also looking forward to reading your thoughts.

PLEASE REVIEW THIS BOOK

ABOUT THE AUTHOR

I. R. Wright was married in 2017. She has one child and lives in a small town outside of New York City where she was also born and raised. This is her first book.

Join the Mailing List:

Irwright.com

Facebook.com/YoungDumbDating

Instagram: @YoungDumbDating

Amazon Author Page

Email: book@youngdumbdating.com